Losing Weight By Burning Fat Rapidly

Healthy and Balanced Lifestyle

This book is a work of non-fiction. Any resemblance to actual people, places, or events is coincidental.

Published by Crown Publishers

Contents

Why Burning Fat Is Important

It is no secret that burning fat is an important part of a healthy lifestyle. Burning fat not only helps to reduce body fat and maintain a healthy weight, but it also has many other benefits such as improved heart health, increased energy levels, and even improved mental health.

For those looking to lose weight, burning fat is the most effective way to do so. When you burn fat, your body is converting stored fat into usable energy. This provides your body with the energy it needs to function and helps to reduce your overall body fat percentage.

The best way to burn fat is through a combination of diet and exercise. Eating a healthy diet that is low in sugar and processed carbohydrates can help to reduce the amount of fat your body stores. Exercise, such as strength training and cardiovascular activities, is essential for burning fat. These activities help to increase your metabolism, which in turn burns more fat.

In addition to diet and exercise, there are several other ways to burn fat. Intermittent fasting is a popular method of burning fat. This involves cycling between periods of eating and fasting, allowing the body to use stored fat for energy. Another popular method of burning fat is through the use of thermogenic supplements. These supplements increase your body temperature, which in turn helps to burn fat more efficiently.

It is important to note that burning fat should be done in a healthy, balanced way. Eating a healthy diet and exercising regularly are key components of a healthy lifestyle and should be done in conjunction with any fat burning methods. It is also important to stay hydrated and get enough sleep. Additionally, consistent and regular exercise is key to burning fat; doing sporadic activity will not be as effective.

Burning fat is an important part of a healthy lifestyle and can have many benefits. Eating a healthy diet and exercising regularly are essential for burning fat, and there are several other methods, such as intermittent fasting and thermogenic supplements, which can help to increase your fat burning potential. It is important to remember that burning fat should be done in a safe and healthy way in order to maximize the benefits.

Definition of metabolism

Metabolism is the process by which our bodies convert food and other substances into energy. It is an important part of our overall health, as it helps to regulate our weight, maintain energy levels, and keep our hormones in check. Without a healthy metabolism, our bodies wouldn't be able to perform many of the essential functions that keep us healthy and functioning.

The metabolism is made up of two parts: catabolism and anabolism. Catabolism is the process by which our bodies break down food into usable energy. This energy is then used to power our cells, providing us with the energy we need to perform everyday tasks. Anabolism is the opposite process, which involves the synthesis of molecules from smaller molecules.

The metabolism is regulated by hormones, and the rate at which our metabolism functions can be affected by certain lifestyle factors such as stress, diet, and exercise. When our bodies are in a state of homeostasis, our metabolism is working efficiently and our weight and energy levels are balanced.

In addition to controlling our weight and energy levels, the metabolism also plays a role in other bodily functions. It helps to regulate our body temperature, convert food into energy, and synthesize proteins, fats, and carbohydrates. It's also responsible for eliminating toxins from the body and maintaining healthy skin, hair, and nails.

Maintaining a healthy metabolism is essential for overall health and wellness. Eating a balanced diet, exercising regularly, and getting enough sleep are all important for keeping the metabolism functioning properly. Additionally, reducing stress and avoiding unhealthy habits such as smoking and drinking can also help to keep the metabolism running smoothly.

Learning more about the metabolism and how it works can help us to better understand our bodies and how to keep them healthy. By making lifestyle changes to support a healthy metabolism, we can ensure that our bodies are functioning at their best.

INTRODUCTION

What if I told you, you could burn fat 24 hours a day?

What if you combined this all day fat burning with the perfect style of cardio and strength training to also shred your fat and maximize your metabolism?

How do you think you would end up looking? How quickly do you think you could get into the top shape of your life?

If your answers to these questions have excited you, I'm here with great news.

YOU can burn fat 24 hours a day. The perfect way to compliment this 24 hour fat burning with cardio and strength training is also available. And the secrets to both these earth shattering revelations are here in this Guide.

Put them into action combined with the rest of the methods I'm about to share with you and you will end up looking your best. And it will happen at a fast and furious pace!

Unless you have a medical disorder which prevents you from getting lean (which is very unlikely) you've been handed a clear plan, that works if you have the will to work it, the fortitude to build the new you.

It's all about mastering your metabolism. Which is the key to learning how to burn fat 24 hours a day.

Here's some of the things that we're going to cover:

Diet Tips And Tricks To Burn Fat 24 Hours A Day.

There's been plenty of things written about diet, some of it worthwhile and some of it worthy of only being ignored. In our Guide you're going to get the most bang for the buck. Strictly what's known and proven to work to super charge your metabolism and get you ripped. With no filler.

Cutting Edge Training Methods To Maximize Metabolism And Look Great.

After diet how your exercise is vitally important. Your training should be helping boost your metabolism, NOT slowing it down. We'll make sure of that.

Supplement Strategies That Can Help The Fight Against Fat.

Don't make any mistake if you know how to filter out misinformation, there are many hugely powerful supplements that can not only burn fat, but also give you added energy when you need it. The secret is knowing what to take and when. And making sure that your safety always come first.

The Lifestyle Choices That Bring All Your Efforts Together And Guarantee Success.

Getting fit and staying fit is all about lifestyle change and choices. With the right plan this doesn't have to be difficult, but it does have to be disciplined. The plan here in our Guide has worked again and again. It will work for

you too, if you apply it!

You're holding in your hands the key to unlocking your metabolism and using it to help reveal your ideal body. A body that looks great, is packed with energy and feels like it's in its prime regardless of your age. These methods work equally well for men and women, the young and old.

When we're done you'll have the equivalent of a Master's degree in metabolism. And be ready and set to burn fat 24 hours a day!

Thanks for giving me the chance to share this knowledge with you.

Benefits of mastering your metabolism

Do you ever feel like you're trying your best to stay healthy, but you just can't seem to make any progress? If so, you may need to take a closer look at your metabolism. The metabolic rate is a complex system responsible for converting food into energy, and when it's not working properly, it can wreak havoc on your health. Fortunately, mastering your metabolism can be a relatively simple process, and the benefits can be enormous.

When it comes to your metabolism, exercise is key. Regular physical activity helps to boost your metabolic rate, so it's important to find an exercise routine that works for you. It doesn't have to be anything extreme; just a few days of moderate physical activity each week can make a big difference. In addition to exercise, it's important to focus on eating nutrient-dense meals. Eating a balanced diet filled with fresh fruits and vegetables can help to give your metabolism the fuel it needs to run efficiently.

It's also important to reduce stress when it comes to mastering your metabolism. Chronic stress can actually result in a reduction in metabolic rate, so it's important to find ways to relax. Mindful meditation, yoga, and other relaxation techniques can help to reduce stress levels and can have a positive impact on your metabolism.

Finally, it's essential to get plenty of sleep. When you don't get enough sleep, your hormones can become imbalanced, which can have an adverse effect on your metabolism. Establishing a consistent sleep schedule and avoiding caffeine and other electronics before bed can help to ensure you get the rest you need.

Mastering your metabolism is an important part of achieving optimal health. Regular exercise, eating nutrient-dense meals, reducing stress, and getting plenty of sleep can all help to boost your metabolic rate. By taking the time to focus on your metabolism, you can reap the many benefits of a healthy, balanced system.

write a powerful and creative article explaining and elucidating   Tips for maintaining a healthy metabolism '

Maintaining a healthy metabolism is essential to feeling your best and having the energy to live your life. Unfortunately, many people struggle with this due to poor diet, lack of exercise, and high levels of stress. Although it may seem daunting to make such drastic lifestyle changes, it's not impossible. Here are a few tips for maintaining a healthy metabolism.

First and foremost, exercise is key to improving metabolism. Regular physical activity helps to speed up the metabolism and increase energy levels. Aim for at least 30 minutes of exercise five days a week. This could include anything from running, biking, swimming, or even just taking a walk.

In addition to exercise, it's important to watch what you eat. Focus on nutrient-dense meals that are filled with vitamins and minerals. This means loading up on fruits, vegetables, and lean proteins. Avoid processed foods and sugary snacks that are high in calories and low in nutrition.

Stress is another factor that can take a toll on your metabolism. Too much stress can cause the body to produce cortisol, which can lead to weight gain and fatigue. Combat stress with mindful meditation, yoga, and other relaxation techniques.

Finally, make sure to get plenty of sleep. Establishing a consistent sleep schedule can help to regulate metabolism and keep energy levels up. Avoid caffeine and electronics at least an hour before bedtime to ensure a good night's sleep.

By following these tips, you can maintain a healthy metabolism and enjoy all the benefits that come with it. Exercise regularly, eat nutrient-dense meals, reduce stress, and get plenty of sleep. With a little effort, you can master your metabolism and feel your best.

METABOLISM 101

Before we dig into how we can turn our bodies into a 24 hour fat burning machine, it's helpful to have an understanding of how metabolism works. Welcome to Metabolism 101. Try to pay attention!

All About Energy

Our bodies are always using energy. We use energy when we run, when we sit behind a computer screen and type, when we do a set of pushups, when we have sex. No matter what we do our body needs to raise up enough energy to perform the function. This is an inescapable fact of life, for better or for worse.

We can split the things that our body does that require energy into two broad categories. The first is automatic functions. The second are functions we choose to perform.

Some examples of automatic functions include our

beating hearts, when our eyes twitch, the working of our livers and kidneys. We don't control any of these, but as we will see later in our Guide dietary and lifestyle choices can certainly affect how much energy we expend on them.

The functions we choose to perform include absolutely everything else we do in our daily lives. Walk the dog? Or get up to grab the milk? No matter what we "do", it requires some sort of energy expenditure.

All this energy is measured in a unit I'm fairly certain you are familiar with the unit. It's called a calorie. Metabolism is defined as "the caloric sum of both your automatic and voluntary functions that must take place in order for the energy forming process to occur."

Metabolism can be broken down into four parts for our purposes here. They are:

1. Resting Metabolic Rate (RMR). This is, by far, the largest part of our metabolism. It counts for over 75% of our daily calorie expenditure. This is where the energy for all of our automatic body functions comes from. Can you

see where even small enhancements here can add up to more pounds of fat lost week after week?

2. Thermal Effect of Feeding (TEF). This is the amount of calories we spend on storing, digesting and absorbing food.

3. Thermal Effect of Activity (TEA). The TEA is the area we can exert the most influence on. It's the amount of calories we spend on activities like cardio and doing strength training. For some of us it can amount to up to 30% of our caloric expenditure a day.

4. Adaptive Thermogenisis (AT). We can think of this as our bodies "adaptive" metabolism. It adjusts up and down based on changes in our environment. Things as varied as the temperature we are operating in to our mental state can affect

AT. This is an area that can be greatly influenced to our fat burning benefit using the secrets you are about to learn in our Guide!

These four pillars of metabolism are usually the enemies of the multitude of us who are trying to look our best and be healthy. We're going to do our best to make them

allies as we learn to burn fat 24 hours a day. The results far exceed the effort!

DIET COMES FIRST

When it comes to mastering your metabolism it should come as no surprise that diet comes first. It comes second and third too! Making smart changes to your diet is the quickest way to start shifting your metabolic gears in favor of burning fat fast.

Follow these tips and no matter where your metabolism is now, it will quickly adjust to where you'd like it to be.

Stay at a Caloric Deficit.

The first pillar of a successful diet plan is to be sure that you're not overeating calories. Now before you get nervous, this doesn't involve you having to do much math at all. Instead we're borrowing an old trick used by bodybuilding and fitness enthusiasts. Take your weight, in pounds, and multiply it by 10. This is the area you want to keep your calorie consumption in.

If you weigh 220lbs that means you will eat 2200 calories a day. 175lbs? 1750 calories a day. It doesn't get much simpler than that.

Never Let Yourself Go Hungry.

Now this may come as a shock, but to keep your body's metabolism burning, it is very important to eat often.

There's no quicker way to cause your metabolism to shut down then to start starving yourself. Your body shifts into a low metabolic state when you go for longer periods of time without eating as a survival mechanism. Unless you use some fairly complicated dietary strategies when this happens you will retain fat. You may even pack more on as you lose muscle!

Your goal is going to be to eat five or six meals a day, but to still eat in the area of your caloric number we determined above. By never getting hungry you are also setting the mental stage to be able to maintain our fat loss program. Believe me, experience has shown personally and with successful clients that if you avoid the feeling of restriction day in and day out you are much more likely to stick with any diet. This one included.

The net caloric deficit will make sure you are losing weight. Your metabolism being high from eating five or six meals a day will aid the fight to be fit by taking off extra fat all day everyday.

Eat The Same Meals Often.

If you're worried about having to count calories to keep yourself in the fat burning zone, there's an easy solution. Eat the same meals often. This removes over thinking the diet and impulse eating. I'd suggest coming up with two or three breakfast, lunch and dinner options. Rotate them as necessary to avoid being bored. No this isn't eating whatever you'd like. But it is a diet that will quickly get you the body of your dreams!

Pick A Free Day.

One day a week eat anything you choose, within reason. Not only will this keep you sane, but it will act as an extra safety net in making sure your metabolism hasn't frozen. Sundays seem to be the favorite choice of many, but pick any day that best fits your schedule. Only eating clean six days a week reaffirms that this is an eating plan that doesn't require an iron discipline to follow. You always have Sunday to look forward to!

Follow these four tips and you will be amazed at how fast the fat melts away. Are you ready to give it a shot?

SPECIFIC FOOD CHOICES TO BOOST YOUR METABOLISM

Good news! Not only can we burn extra fat based on how much we eat and when we eat it, we can also help boost our metabolism by choosing to eat specific foods.

The principal is to avoid as much processed foods as possible. The things you'll find on the list that follow taste great and all have fat burning properties. Incorporate them into your diet and the fat burning flames will burn higher and brighter!

Salmon.

The overall health benefits of Omega 3 fatty acids are pretty remarkable. Among them is that they help optimize metabolism. There's hardly a better whole food choice of Omega 3's than salmon. The combination of healthy protein and fats can't be beat. Eat salmon as often as you are able.

Eat Organic Fruit And Vegetables With Edible Skin.

Yes, going "all organic" can be expensive. On a budget the best thing you can do for your metabolism is to at least try to go with organic veggies with edible skin. This includes tomatoes, cucumbers, green beans, apples and pears. The skin of these fruits and vegetables free of harmful chemicals augments your metabolism rather than slows it down. The more you eat, especially of the organic vegetables, the better. Aim for three servings a day as a bare minimum.

Yogurt.

Now please understand, this doesn't mean the style of yogurt that comes packed with sugary fruit on the bottom, but instead plain (preferably organic) yogurt. Yogurt again provides us with much needed protein, but is also packed with probiotics which not only help the digestive process, fight belly fat, but some scientists also say boosts metabolism. Eat more yogurt and get the flat stomach you've been dreaming of. Makes both a great breakfast and snack choice.

Avocado

One of the enemies of a fast metabolism is inflammation. No common food fights inflammation as well as avocado. Add avocado to your salads, as a side with your dinner and as a snack in the form of guacamole. In addition to its inflammation fighting power avocado is packed with fiber, which will go a long way in helping you feel full even while you're eating smaller meals. Try for one serving a day.

Chili Peppers.

If you love hot food you are in luck! Chili peppers give a huge boost to metabolism. Now I understand they aren't for all of us, but if you enjoy (or can tolerate) the taste dig in. The best choices include jalapeno, chipolte and habanero, along with Thai peppers. The hotter the better!

Beans.

Inexpensive and high in fiber beans are an ideal choice to make your body burn more calories day in and out. They are near perfect for boosting metabolism and should become a constant companion with all of your major meals. Recent research points to the starch in beans causing a 25% jump in energy expenditure during the digestion process. Remember, this ends up equally less calories that you have to worry about burning through other means which can be a real blessing.

Coffee.

Great for energy and excellent for your metabolism. Just be sure you don't make it into a calorie packed monstrosity. Go black with stevia for sweetness and keep it simple. Coffee will likely be your best friend as you work your way through our Guide! The more energy we have the more we can get done, after all.

This shouldn't be considered an exclusive list of metabolic boosting foods, just a good starting point. Feel free to research and explore!

SMART CARDIO TO KEEP THE FIRE BURNING

Cardio is the art and science of burning calories. As a nice side effect it will also help make you healthier and more able to perform things you enjoy. These range from sports, to play, to making love. Increase your ability to do cardio and your whole life is enhanced. One of the best parts of this is what happens when you do cardio the RIGHT way: your metabolism is enhanced to the point where you not only burn calories while you train, but continue burning them for the rest of the day too!

Why the emphasis on the "right" kind of cardio? Well all cardio will knock off calories. But not all cardio is ideal for boosting your all day metabolism. In fact some of it, like long distance marathon running, is even bad for it.

Smart Cardio Tips to Keep the Fire Burning

You Pick Your Cardio Choice.

There's plenty of ways to get in your cardio. Running, biking and using a rowing machine are just a few examples. Pick whichever you enjoy most and work best with your lifestyle. As long as you are sweating and breathing hard your choice will do the job!

Do Your Cardio Five Days a Week.

To get the most out of cardio you need to do it often. Five or even six days a week are optimal. If this leaves you too sore early into your training start off with four days until your body's endurance grows. One or two days of cardio a week will not do anything for your metabolism at all. No one said getting the body of your dreams would be easy.

HIIT Your Cardio Hard.

The style of cardio which is the absolute best for cutting fat and boosting your metabolism is called High Intensity

Interval Training or HIIT for short. Whole books have been written on the subject, but here it is in a nutshell. Your cardio will be intense with a recovery period mixed in, in short training sessions.

Here's an example using running on a treadmill, but the same principle can be used for other methods depending on what you choose to do: 30 seconds of all out running (think of an 8 to 10 difficulty level) followed by light jogging for 1 minute (think a 3 or 4 difficulty). Repeat these HIIT "sets" for 15 minutes. As you become more fit up the total workout sessions to 20, 25 and finally 30 minutes. If you've never trained HIIT style be prepared to see results very, very quickly.

Don't Miss Training Sessions.

To boost metabolism consistent cardio training is what we are looking for. This requires a commitment to do your HIIT sessions and not let small things get in your way.

Work late? Do your cardio afterwards. Feel under the weather? Drink some coffee and break a sweat. The willingness to train despite obstacles that may appear is one of the things that separate the people who achieve their dream bodies and those who remain fat and lacking in health. Be a winner and don't miss training sessions.

Consider these tips the Holy Grail of metabolic boosting cardio training. Take action and incorporate them in your program and your body will look and feel better. Are you ready to make that kind of change?

FULL BODY BLASTS TO BURN EVEN MORE FAT

Muscle is the best friend of a high metabolism.

This may come as a surprise to you in a Guide about losing fat and getting lean, but it's one of the most important secrets I have to share.

Strength training is a vital component of making sure your body is burning fat 24 hours a day. Every pound of muscle you put on will help you lose two pounds of fat. And a certain style of strength training will absolutely crank up your metabolism into overdrive. Putting in the effort to get stronger will also get you leaner and healthier too. All this combined will have you looking your absolute best before you know it.

So here's how to train to get lean. You'll be doing full body blasts three days a week.

- Pick Three Non-Consecutive Days to Train.

I like Monday, Wednesday and Friday. Your choice will likely be influenced by your work or school schedule, but three days a week is a must.

- Each Day You Will be Doing Full Body Workouts.

- You'll Need a Barbell and two Dumbbells at the Least.

If you are training in a gym this is certainly available. If not pick yourself up an inexpensive set, along with a reasonable amount tof weight plates. It's a worthy investment that will last forever.

- You can Strength Train Before or After Your Cardio Session.

Whichever choice works best for your lifestyle is fine. Just don't neglect either, they are both of vital importance in optimizing your metabolism.

- Do Three Sets of 15 reps for Each Exercise.

- Alternate Between Each Exercise after Each set.

When all three sets are done move on to the next two exercises and follow the same method.

Pair 1

- Barbell Squat. Place barbell with weights across shoulders, squat down to just below parallel. Always squat in a rack or with a spotter.

- Dumbbell Rows. Put one knee on bench hold dumbbell in opposite hand. Pull dumbbell to core. This works the middle back.

Pair 2

- Pushups. These should be performed with tight abs and back using strict form.

- Situps. Bent knee situps or crunches. If you can do more than 15 reps do so.

Pair 3

- Pull Downs or Pullups. Both are fine upper back and overall strength building exercises. If you are able choose pullups over machine pull downs. There's a reason they are the favorite exercise of athletes and the military.

- Bicep Curls. These can be done with either a barbell, with dumbbells or even on a machine.

Pair 4

- Dead Lift. Load a barbell on the floor. Bend your knees and pull the bar up to the middle quad as you straighten your legs. This builds total body strength. It is also credited by many trainers as offering a total body metabolic boost.

- Leg Lifts. Lie on your back and raise your straight legs to the sky stopping at the "L" point. This builds the lower and side abdominal muscles.

Being strong and being lean and fit all come hand in hand. If you would like more information on technique or correct form for exercises listed above please do a search online, there is lots of great videos and step by step instructions.

Dedicate yourself to this full body blast strength training even for a month and watch the new you burst through! Don't be surprised if it becomes your favorite part of the program.

FOUR SUPPLEMENTS YOU CAN'T DO WITHOUT

I can't stress enough that the subject of supplements needs to be approached with caution. But probably not for the reason you think. Nearly all the supplements on the market today are relatively safe, so if you thought it was a health concern with supplementation you're wrong. What we need to avoid is the many "miracle" promising fat loss pills and powders that are nothing but marketing schemes. The only thing these supplements will make thinner is your wallet!

These four supplements are the exact opposite of what's offered by those looking for a quick buck. They work well and if you choose to add them to your daily regime they will boost your metabolism and give you a significant edge in burning fat. Check them out.

Caffeine.

There was a time years ago when a great many "thermogenic" supplements were on the market. Many worked incredibly well, but were so abused they ended up being banned in most countries. Now these banned supplements have been replaced with products with similar names but which contain, for the most part, caffeine.

This isn't a bad thing. Caffeine is safe, when taken in reasonable doses, boosts metabolism and can give a much needed charge for your training sessions. My suggestion - skip the bottles with the fancy names and instead buy caffeine pills which are marketed for fat loss.

You'll get the same dose and they are usually about 75% less expensive. A good dose? Depending on your tolerance and bodyweight this

will vary, but for most people 200mg twice a day
is a good start.

Zinc.

Recent studies have revealed a large percentage of athletes who are having trouble shedding weight are suffering from a zinc deficiency. It seems hard training

can even cause this shortage of zinc to occur quickly, making it an area where dietary problems can manifest even in those who are making a point of breaking a sweat everyday. Zinc will not only help optimize your metabolism and speed up recovery time, it will also help you get a great night's sleep. Take 15mg a day right before bed.

Carnitine.

Carnitine is an essential amino acid, which carries a great weight in how active your metabolism will be. It's available in large doses in red meat, which means if you are vegan or vegetarian you have a great chance of not taking in enough carnitine everyday. Supplement with a gram a day divided in to two or three doses. A nice added bonus of supplementing with carnitine is the added energy it also brings. You may have noticed it as an ingredient in things like Red Bull for just this reason.

Green Tea Extract.

Drinking green tea is excellent for your metabolism and taking green tea extract is even better. At 300mg a day

green tea extract is a very powerful fat burner which will help keep you in the fat burning zone all day and night. It is also pretty much jitter free. Just be sure to buy from a reputable company. For whatever reason, there's way too many junk green tea supplements on the market in the last few years. I guess we can blame Dr. Oz for making it so popular!

These four supplements are worth their weight in gold. And they won't break the bank. Try them and see what you think.

THE SECRET OF STRETCHING

Now we're entering an area that's skipped by nearly every mainstream book that looks at boosting metabolism. I know because I've read dozens of them.

It's a shame too, because it's easy, it works and not only will it help you get leaner, but it will also protect you against injury. So for now it's a secret only known by a chosen few.

It's stretching and it's effect on metabolism and weight loss. I use the word stretching to not scare off anyone, but if you feel more comfortable you could also use the term Yoga. The choice is yours!

Here's what I've learned and why you should stretch everyday without fail:

Stretching Improves Digestion.

Poor digestive function and a liver which isn't operating well will slow down your metabolism without fail. Full body stretching which includes things like hand to toe stretched (standing and sitting) will act to reinvigorate your digestive process. This quickly leads to an increased metabolism as your body more efficiently eliminates toxins.

Stretching Will Build Eye Appealing Muscle.

Stretching helps build stronger and more visually appealing muscle. This added muscle, like we've touched on earlier, will boost your metabolism even further. For my women readers, this isn't "huge" bodybuilding muscle, but it builds a toned and strong natural looking physique nearly everyone admires.

Stretching Enhances Circulation.

If you are experiencing circulation issues, which you may be without even realizing it, they are also likely to be causing your metabolism to be sluggish.

Can you see how metabolism is a whole body concern? Getting your circulation flowing well again comes quickly with daily stretching sessions. For those into Eastern mysticism this circulation increase also serves to open up the body's chakras and internal energy movement. The end result is looking and feeling better.

Stretching Helps Prevent Overeating.

Stretching will work perfectly with your practice of eating multiple small meals in keeping extreme hunger away.

Many clients have even found that a quick stretching session works to kill hunger when they are being faced with irritating food cravings. How's that for a healthy appetite suppressant?

Learning to Stretch

Intrigued, but unfamiliar with how to stretch or do Yoga? Don't worry the learning curve for basic stretches is very small. I'd suggest you take these steps:

Ask A Friend For Instruction.

Most of us know someone who does Yoga. Ask them to come by and teach you some basic stretches to do every morning. You can easily learn them in a few hours.

Join A Yoga School.

Yoga and Pilates schools are everywhere. Many are very inexpensive. Stop by a school, take a class and help your metabolism. You may even greatly expand your positive social circle in the process!

Watch Videos.

While it is very difficult to teach stretches or Yoga from a distance, places like YouTube and Vimeo do offer some really awesome videos which can both help you learn and provide inspiration. Do a search and see what's being offered.

Your body burning fat 24 hours a day is a sign of vibrant health. Stretching is one of the ways to build that health. Flexibility and fat loss are two awesome things, so dive in with enthusiasm!

THE MIND AND METABOLISM

Losing weight is never just a physical thing. In fact for a great many people the physical part comes pretty easily. They can do their cardio, hit the gym even eat right.

Where they end up losing out, is when their mind gives in.

Getting lean is probably at least 75% mental. Maybe more. The mind and metabolism are linked whether we like it or not.

Once we accept this fact, we need to start working on doing everything we can to getting our mind on board with our body becoming a 24 hour fat burning machine. It can happen if you follow these tips. And please know once your mind and body are working in the same direction, absolutely anything, and I mean ANYTHING, is possible!

Think Positive.

You may be under the misconception that positive thinking is just some kind of "new age" fad, but it's anything but that.

Your mind can be rightly thought of as the general or coach of your body. When it thinks negative and defeatist thoughts you sap yourself of energy, and studies have even shown, slow down your metabolism. That's right, negative can make you or keep you fat. By simply forcing yourself to consider positive spins on situations when you find your thoughts getting "dark" you can break this cycle.

It's hard at first for most people. Within 30 days of doing it, it becomes a habit. Wouldn't you rather have this habit that works for you, over ones that harm you for a change?

Affirm Fitness.

Cut out some photos of people who possess the type of body you are striving for. Or they could even be of a younger and fitter you. Place these where you will see them often. Like your bathroom mirror, in your car and especially on your refrigerator. This keeps your mind focused on your body goals and makes pigging out much more difficult to do. The trick is to look at them often and remind yourself, in a way that's charged with emotion, how happy you will be once you meet these fitness goals.

Learn To Calm Your Mind.

Many people over eat as a means to fight anxiety. This is something over eating is remarkably bad at, considering the end result (becoming over weight) just adds another issue to be anxious about. Rather than replacing over eating with some other vice (like alcohol or drugs), consider adding a short nightly meditation session to your program. This doesn't have to be even remotely

complicated. Sitting and focusing on your breath, with eyes shut in silence for ten minutes works brilliantly to decompress the mind. If this approach appeals to you pursue meditation training further. It could change your life,

Reward Your Wins.

Reinforcing your positive behavior goes a long way towards continuing it. Getting lean and fit can be hard work, even when you are burning fat 24 hours a day. If you've hit one of your goals on the scale or in the mirror make a point of rewarding yourself. Maybe get that new outfit you couldn't fit in last year without looking ridiculous, or spend a night out with your partner.

Regardless, make sure you reward yourself for doing the right thing. This will help keep that positive momentum going!

Your mind can be the best of allies. Cultivate that relationship!

CRITICAL MISTAKES THAT NEED TO BE AVOIDED

Now that we have an understanding of what you should be doing, for your sanity's sake it makes good sense to go over what you SHOULDN'T be doing too. These are critical mistakes I've seen friends and clients make when attempting to amp up their metabolism and get lean. I've even made some of them myself.

Keep an eye out for these things. If you see them it's a good idea to correct them QUICKLY. If not you run the risk of seeing your plan not succeed as well as you would like. Or possibly not at all.

Not Eating Frequently Enough.

To keep your metabolism's flames burning you need to be eating five or six times a day. Cutting calories alone is not enough. If you aren't losing weight despite cutting

calories and see you are only eating two or three times a day it's clear your metabolism is slowing down. Eat more frequently and make metabolism your friend! This is probably the number one mix up made by people trying out our program here and having difficulties.

Eating Too Many Calories.

This is our second most common mistake. If you aren't losing weight write down EVERYTHING you eat or drink for three days and see if some hidden calories you didn't calculate managed to sneak in. If you still can't find anything cut your calories by an additional 10% and stick with the program.

Using this method will either find the problem or bring your calories down to a point where you are burning calories like wildfire again!

Going Heavy On Carbohydrates After Lunch.

Carbohydrates are fuel. When this fuel isn't used it becomes, for the most part, fat. Eating large amounts of

carbohydrates, not burning them off, and then going to sleep is a recipe for disaster. For most of us that means keep the carbs low after lunch unless we train later in the evening. When do you eat most of your carbs?

Expecting Your Supplements To Be A Magic Bullet.

They aren't. Yes, they'll help if you take the ones we have mentioned here in our Guide and you use them smartly.

But if you are thinking they will perform miracles, rest assured they won't. Getting the body of your dreams requires work and discipline. Whoever tries to tell you it doesn't is likely trying to sell you something, so be very suspicious.

Not Drinking Enough Water.

Dehydration is the enemy of a quick metabolism. You should be drinking near a gallon of clean, pure water a day. Including at least half a litre right when you wake up in the morning. If you let yourself get dehydrated too frequently it can take a week of re-hydration to normalize your body system before any of your work on boosting your metabolism even really starts to take hold. When in doubt, drink more water.

Of course there's other mistakes too. But keeping these in mind and correcting them as they appear will put you way ahead of the pack. Knowledge is power!

PUTTING IT ALL TOGETHER - AN ACTION PLAN

Now you have a proven program to get the most out of your body. What do you plan to do with it?

The sad truth is over 70% of readers, if the statistics are to be believed, will do absolutely nothing.

Don't be one of those people!

Taking action is the most important thing you can do right now. Consider these suggestions your official Action Plan!

Start Right NOW.

The most important thing you can do to make sure you follow through with the information you have just taken the time and made the effort to learn is to take

IMMEDIATE action. Immediate as in right now. Make an immediate change to your eating patterns, start your cardio and begin doing some strength training. Every day you put it off makes it much more likely you won't EVER make a real
drive towards changing your body for the better.

* Write Down Your Long and Short Term Goals. Having clear goals makes success come much, much easier. Set your long term goal of what you'd like to look like and weigh (which is a quantifiable number that lets you set as a target) as well as continually updated weekly goals. For your weekly goals I'd suggest to not focus so much on the scale, but rather on how many training sessions you will engage in and other motivating, achievable, set points. Goal setting is a skill that can revolutionize your entire life, including your fitness plans. The more you put into this important area, the more it will reward you.

Food Shop In Bulk.

The less you go to the store to shop, the less likely you are to impulse buy junk food. A better method is to shop

once a week with a list in hand get done and get out. If you aren't around food that will wreck your diet, you won't eat it. It's a fact that's hard to argue with.

Get A Training Partner.

Studies have shown those of us who train with a partner are much more inclined to stick with our training and diet plans. Maybe it's because we are social animals at heart or maybe it's our competitive nature. Regardless of the reason take advantage of this truth and get a training partner if you can. If it's someone who lives in your household it's even better. Having someone to achieve your dream body with makes for an adventure the two of you can share with others for years to come!

Don't Give Up.

Every person who puts in the time and work to get fit ends up hitting some speed bumps along the way. It could be a loss of motivation, a small injury or social problems with friends who aren't quite ready to give up

the "fat" you. Rise above these obstacles. Not giving up is what separates those who "can" from those who "could", but didn't. The struggles along the way will make everything much more worthwhile in the end. If it was easy, it wouldn't be an adventure!

Thank you for joining me on this wild adventure of learning how to make metabolism a friend and not a foe. I have no doubt you will use this information to forge the new you. I can't wait to hear about your results!

Frequently Asked Questions

Question: I really enjoyed running marathons about a decade ago, but since then I've packed on the pounds. Is it okay for me to follow your suggestions, but to do marathon training rather than the cardio solutions you suggest?

Answer: Great question! If you'd like to train for marathons you can, of course. But I'd suggest you lose the extra weight first using HIIT and once you are leaner and build up your strength then make the switch to long distance low intensity cardio work that marathon training requires. That type of training can kill your metabolism and make it very hard to quickly lose weight, so lose the weight first. But certainly any activity is better than no activity so whatever you choose to do, make sure it involves getting off the couch!

Question: I'm pretty caffeine sensitive. What do you think I should use to help boost metabolism if caffeine really isn't an option?

Answer: Caffeine free Green Tea extract is a perfect choice for you. You'll not get the jitters, but you'll still have some of the metabolic boost of the caffeine based thermogenics. This route may even, ultimately, be a healthier option for many people, especially those in their 40's and beyond.

Question: I hate breakfast. Can I skip it and still optimize my metabolism?

Answer: Well, you can certainly not eat a traditional breakfast in the form of eggs and bacon or cereal or whatever. But you will still need to get in some calories. I'd suggest a protein shake or smoothie, which will serve the same purpose, is quick to put together and you can even drink it in the car on the way to work or school if you need to!

Question: Can prescription medications effect metabolism?

Answer: Yes, of course they can. Most hurt, but some can

actually help. I'd suggest discussing with your doctor the effects of any medications you are on and getting his (or her) opinion. Your health should always come first, so never discontinue an important medication without clearing it with your health care professional first. No diet is worth risking your safety for!

Question: How long will the suggestions in the Guide work for? Will I eventually need to switch them up to get my metabolism raging again?

Answer: These tips will work as long as you work them. I purposely left out any short term fixes and focused all the content here on real solutions that will work for most people over the long haul. This is how you can establish healthy habits that you can count on over a lifetime. Diets that are short term fixes can serve a purpose in certain circumstances, but what you have here is fitness gold thats built to last.

Question: I'd like to follow this plan while I continue to train at my local CrossFit club. How well do you think the two go with each other?

Answer: For the more athletically minded CrossFit and similar programs make an awesome mix with our program in this Guide. If you haven't noticed they use full body workouts and cardio sessions that are very HIIT friendly. So go for it! The results will be awesome!